Aromatic Immunity: Navigating Essential Oil Research for Cancer, Autoimmune, and Chronic Inflammatory Conditions

Amy Kreydin

The Barefoot Dragonfly LLC

Austin, Texas 78729

http://www.thebarefootdragonfly.com

ISBN: 978-1987698121
ASIN B07B2F7VKD

"I go to nature to be soothed and healed and to have my senses put in order."

– John Burroughs

Introduction

The immune system is a fascinating network of organs, tissues, cells, and molecules that protect us from infection, heal wounds, and keep us healthy. Dysregulation can occur from external and internal stressors, causing the immune system to under or over perform. Aromatherapy, my beloved modality, can be used to soothe chronic inflammation, support healthy lifestyle practices that prevent cancer, and ease emotional wounds that negatively influence immunity. The practice of aromatherapy is holistic by design and backed by the modern science of aromatic chemistry as well as the ancient healing arts that have been passed down to us for thousands of years.

As a teenager I was captivated by the healing arts and spent years studying and observing my mentors in Native American healing, Latin folk healing (called *curanderismo*), faith healing, midwifery, Western herbal medicine, permaculture, Ayurveda, ancient Greek and Perso-Arabic medicine, traditional Chinese medicine, and horticulture. Later, I trained in reflexology, a therapeutic bodywork modality which theorizes that the entire body is interconnected and that specific pressure techniques applied to one part of the body can cause a response in another part. Autoimmunity, specifically multiple sclerosis, was the subject of my research paper, my case studies giving me firsthand insight into how the body can be gently nudged into healing after months or years of destroying healthy cells and tissues. After a summer of reflexology sessions, one of my case studies resumed walking for the first time in seven years. Another case study was able to return to driving when the neuropathy in her feet and lower legs resolved.

My studies in clinical aromatherapy brought my education back to my roots in botanical medicine. In my studio here in Central Texas, my apothecary cabinets and cold storage house a wide variety of aromatics. I'll be sharing some of the following with you throughout this book:

- essential oils – featuring hundreds of volatile chemical constituents in each bottle, are obtained through steam and water distillation of seeds, bark, resins, leaves, flowers, and roots, or via the mechanical-pressing of citrus peels;
- absolutes – delicate flowers like jasmine are submerged in solvent then washed in alcohol to produce heady extracts;
- CO2 extracts – carbon dioxide is used to extract the essential oils (volatiles), fats, waxes, and pigments for an aromatic extract that resembles the plant's overall chemistry and aroma;
- hydrosols – steam is passed through fresh plant material, then quickly chilled to return it to its liquid state, where it holds perfectly suspended micro-droplets of essential oils and the plant's cellular waters;

- resins – dried sap from trees like frankincense, and myrrh are ready to be dissolved in alcohol, burned on charcoal as incense, or infused in fatty lipids for topical or oral dosing;
- aromatic herbs and spices – preserved fresh in alcohol, dried ready for a tea or liniment, or extracted into alcohol.

With this book I hope to bridge the gap of knowledge between the worlds of scientific research and the holistic art of aromatherapy while giving some perspective on how we might approach immune dysregulation. This isn't a book which lists the top essential oils for {insert disease here}, then leaves the reader wondering how to apply the information to their wellness plan. In fact, it challenges the validity of those offering quick cures and blanket claims that could cause very real harm to readers with serious health concerns.

While the book is designed to be read front to back, I anticipated that some may wish to jump straight to sections that apply to themselves or a loved one. For this reason, I have included some information in more than one chapter, especially in cases where an aromatic impacts the immune system in more than one way or if key therapeutic guidelines apply to more than one condition. My hope is that curious aromatic enthusiasts find this volume helpful in answering important questions about aromatic immunity.

In health,

Amy Kreydin, NBCR, CCAP, BD
Board Certified Reflexologist
Clinical Aromatherapy Practitioner
Aromatic Medicine Practitioner
Metamorphic Technique Practitioner
DONA Trained Birth Doula

Contents

PART I: IMMUNOMODULATION AND AROMATICS

1 Aromatics and the Immune System

"To reach the individual we need an individual remedy. Each of us is a unique message. It is only the unique remedy that will suffice. We must, therefore, seek odiferous substances which present affinities with the human being we intend to treat, those which will compensate for his deficiencies and those which will make his faculties blossom." – Marguerite Maury

When it comes to essential oils and the immune system, what we don't know has the potential to harm us more than benefit us. There are plenty of essential oil products on the market promising to *boost immunity*, but there's not a lot of dialogue around whether it is ideal to regularly *stimulate* the immune system. And while there's a ton of websites that promise curative essential oils for cancer, chronic inflammation, and autoimmunity, we don't see them mentioning what the risks of using immune-influencing essential oils are for these conditions.

Somewhere along the way, I feel like aromatic therapies got misrepresented as these all-natural drugs that will cure everything from flu to cancer. The really exciting parts of aromatics got left in the dust, probably owing to the complexity of aromatic chemistry and the practice of holistic medicine that dictates we must understand the nature of the individual before we treat them.

My initial education in aromatic immunity focused mostly on supporting innate immunity through antimicrobial essential oils. In class, my instructor touched on the field of study that looks at psychosomatic processes that influence the immune system, known as psychoneuroimmunology. A few years ago I had a lightbulb (aha!) moment about the depth and breadth of aromatic immunity while conversing with Robert Tisserand, co-author of Essential Oil Safety (2014), on a social media site. The discussion was on persons with autoimmune conditions, and he cited a study on immunostimulating essential oils as a possible caution. It hadn't occurred to me prior to this discussion that any essential oils should be avoided in autoimmunity. I decided to study these potential influences of aromatics on the immune system with multiple anatomy and physiology books and dozens of research studies in tow.

Immunomodulation

Aromatics that are employed in clinical aromatherapy include essential oils, hydrosols, CO2 extracts, resins, and absolutes. There is promising research indicating that some aromatics can have immunomodulatory actions on the immune system (Anastasiou, et al 2017). These unique actions are broken down into how they affect an immune response:

- Attenuation – will have a suppressive action.
- Amplification – will have an enhancing or intensifying action.
- Inducement – will have a stimulating or triggering action.

Each of these distinct actions has their own benefits and risks when we look at therapeutic applications on the immune system of individuals with diverse wellness goals. Attenuation, or suppression of immune response, might be appropriate for someone with a progressive autoimmune condition as part of a wellness plan for remission. Amplification, or intensification of the immune response, would be worth considering for the wellness plan of someone recovering from an illness. Inducement, or stimulation of the immune response, might be indicated for someone who has completed chemotherapy and is on a wellness plan to recover immunity after treatment.

To better understand how aromatics can potentially have these very different actions on the immune system we need to have some background on the physiology of immunity.

Immune System

The immune system is composed of organs, molecules, cells, and a collection of tissues, that work in conjunction to prevent and eradicate infections (Abbas et al 2016). Lymphocytes, a type of white blood cell, are made from the red bone marrow found in the skull, spine, sternum, ribs, clavicle, pelvis, and the ends of the humerus (arm) and femur (leg) bones. Some lymphocytes (B cells like phagocytes and natural killer cells) are matured in the bone marrow, whereas cytotoxic and helper T cells mature in the thymus and are specifically programmed to target substances foreign to the body. A healthy individual will have about a trillion (10^{12}) lymphocytes (Alberts et al., 2002) that circulate in the body's blood and lymph and can be found in the spleen and lymph nodes.

Healthy individuals have two levels of immune defense - innate and adaptive - which assist each other in keeping us well. We're born with innate immunity, which relies on the skin and mucous membranes to act as the first line of defense against microbes. B cell lymphocytes act as mediators, ready to attack in the event that the microbe finds a way past the barriers of the skin and mucous membranes.

Inflammation is an innate immunity response to irritants, injury, and infectious agents (Stevens et al., 2016). We recognize it by its signature symptoms of pain, swelling, heat, and tissue redness. White blood cells known as neutrophils respond to an irritant or pathogen by ingesting it or releasing enzymes that neutralize it. These neutrophils respond to injury by breaking down injured tissue, allowing lymphocytes to come in and remove the waste. We would not be able to heal cuts, scrapes, bruises, and other tissue trauma if we didn't have the innate immune system's proinflammatory response.

Adaptive immunity is something that is developed over time as our immune system responds to foreign particles, allowing for more precision as it recognizes a wider variety of molecules - both infectious and non-infectious. Specialized T cell lymphocytes work against intracellular microbes from the inside. They can kill host cells that have infectious microbes in the cytoplasm or trigger the destruction of microbes that the B cell phagocytes have ingested. T cells use protein antigens to let them know when there is a microbe inside a cell.

T cells are broken down into groups known as Clusters of Differentiation (CD). Types of T cells include:

- Helper – CD4 T cells
- Cytotoxic – CD8 T cells
- Memory – these can be either CD4 or CD8 T cells
- Regulatory (Treg) – CD4 T cells
- Natural Killer (NKT) – natural killer T cells

Disorders and deficiencies within the immune system can leave us vulnerable to illness, chronic inflammation, cancer, and autoimmunity. Researchers have looked at the relationship between one of the regulatory T cells and another T cell that produces a proinflammatory cytokine, interleukin 17 (Th17). These two different cell populations have a lot in common, so they are susceptible to influences from each other. When dysregulated inflammatory conditions like autoimmunity arise, the rejection of skin and tissue grafts, and the formation of tumors can occur (Diller et al., 2016).

Another example is the implication of natural killer T cells in inflammatory processes. NKT cell deficiency may predispose an individual to Lyme disease, some types of cancer, multiple sclerosis, systemic lupus erythematosus, and rheumatoid arthritis (Berzins et al., 2011).

We want the immune system to be able to keep us healthy by being vigilant and protecting us against infections as well as assisting in healing tissue injuries. When external and internal stressors cause it to fail, we end up with a dysregulated immune response that is over or under responsive. In the following chapters we'll explore aromatics than can potentially modulate the immune system. Later, in part two, we'll explore how to integrate these aromatics into wellness plans designed to gently guide the immune system back to homeostasis where health and wellness lie.

2 Immune Stimulating and Amplifying Aromatics

"What a pity flowers can utter no sound! - A singing rose, a whispering violet, a murmuring honeysuckle... oh, what a rare and exquisite miracle would these be!"
- Henry Ward Beecher

Amplifying aromatics have the potential to enhance or intensify the immune response. Stimulating aromatics will have the potential to trigger or induce an immune response. Either of these may have an effect on innate immunity, adaptive immunity, or a bit of both. Some aromatics appear to have amphoteric action, in which they can both stimulate and suppress different parts of the immune system at the same time, and they may have dose dependent actions as well.

This is an exciting and new area of research, and in many cases we don't have human research trials to give us clear guidance on how to effectively dose aromatics for immune modulating behavior. Persons with chronic inflammation and autoimmune conditions may wish to explore how these aromatics affect their immune response. I recommend clients use an *Inflammation Log* (see Appendix A for example) to track positive and negative responses. If exacerbation, recurrence of symptoms, or marked progression occurs, you may wish to discontinue usage of that particular aromatic.

In 2006, Australian researchers published their *in vitro* research in the International Journal of Aromatherapy that looked at whether natural killer cell (NK) and lymphocyte activation occurred with essential oils of German Chamomile (*Matricaria recutita*), Frankincense (*Boswellia carteri*), Geranium (*Pelargonium graveolens*), Lavender (*Lavandula angustifolia*), Lemon (*Citrus limon*), Tea Tree (*Melaleuca alternifolia*), Niaouli (*Melaleuca viridiflora*), Sandalwood (*Santalum spicatum*), Atlas Cedar (*Cedrus atlantica*), and Thyme ct. linalool (*Thymus vulgaris*) (Standen et al., 2006). The study found that natural killer cells, part of the innate immune system, were stimulated by the essential oil constituents of linalyl acetate and trans-caryophyllene (or β-caryophyllene).

Essential oils rich in linalyl acetate include:

- Bergamot, distilled and cold-pressed
- Clary Sage
- Lavandin, Super
- Lavender
- Linaloe, wood
- Petitgrain (Orange leaf Bigarade)

Essential oils rich in β-caryophyllene include:
- Black Pepper
- Catnip
- Copaiba Balsam

In 2014, Italian researchers published *in vitro* findings in the journal *Phytotherapy Research* that showed bergamot essential oil to have proinflammatory action, thought to contribute to this botanical's ability to facilitate wound healing (Consentino et al., 2014).

The same journal published research findings from a group of Argentinian researchers in 2008 that found d-limonene stimulated lymphocyte proliferation (production) and had an antiproliferative action on tumor cells *in vitro* (Manuele et al., 2008).

Essential oils rich in d-limonene include:
- Sweet Orange
- Grapefruit
- Clementine
- Tangerine
- Lemon, cold-pressed and distilled
- Mandarin
- Palo Santo
- Lime, distilled and cold-pressed
- Bergamot, distilled and cold-pressed

Japanese researchers conducted an aromatherapy massage study published in the journal *Evidence-Based Complementary and Alternative Medicine* in 2005 looking at the essential oils of Lavender, Cypress, Sweet Marjoram, and Tea Tree in a massage. The researchers found that cytotoxic (CD8) T cells were increased and that the helper and cytotoxic T cell ratio, CD4/CD8, was significantly reduced in their volunteers (Kuriyama et al., 2005).

University of California researchers published research on mice in *Immunopharmacology* in 1986, finding that the constituent of eugenol had a suppressive action on T cells residing in the spleen (splenocytes) when used at low dose, a total inhibition at high dose, and in both doses 'significantly enhanced' natural killer (NK) cell activity (Vishteh et al., 1986).

Essential oils rich in eugenol include:
- Clove, bud, stem, and leaf
- Cinnamon, leaf
- Pimento, berry and leaf
- Bay, West Indian
- Holy Basil (Tulsi)

List of potential immunostimulating aromatics:

- Basil, Holy (Tulsi)
- Bay, West Indian
- Bergamot, distilled and cold-pressed
- Clementine
- Cinnamon, leaf
- Clove, bud, stem, and leaf
- Cypress
- Grapefruit
- Lavender
- Lemon, cold-pressed and distilled
- Lime, distilled and cold-pressed
- Orange, Sweet
- Mandarin
- Marjoram, Sweet
- Palo Santo
- Pimento, berry and leaf
- Tangerine
- Tea Tree

Oxidized Essential Oils

There have been multiple studies that have looked at the pro-inflammatory action of essential oils when an essential oil has been allowed to oxidize. In a 1992 study published in *Contact Dermatitis*, researchers found that when d-limonene, found mainly in citrus essential oils, was oxidized it became a "potent allergen" (Karlberg et al., 1992). Researcher Mihály Matura, MD, PhD, has published a series of papers on oxidized citrus oil as potential skin sensitizers and contact allergens (Matura 2002, 2006).

Essential oils can cause two different types of allergic reactions: immediate hypersensitivity and delayed hypersensitivity (Tisserand, Young 2014). In the case of the former, the immune system responds to the allergen with a release of white blood cells, known as mast cells, that release histamine and create a localized inflammatory response. This antibody response is usually much larger in comparison to the small concentration of the essential oil. In the case of a delayed reaction, T cells become sensitized following the initial exposure - a process that takes 1-2 weeks. Upon a subsequent exposure, the allergen is presented to the T cells,activating Th1 cells and resulting in an inflammatory response with edema and tissue destruction (Stevens et al., 2016). If the essential oil is oxidized, there is an increased risk of this immune response.

3 Immune Suppressing Aromatics

"We may need to be cured by flowers." – Sharman Apt Russell

Suppressive aromatics have the potential to lessen an immune response by affecting innate immunity, adaptive immunity, or a combination of the two. Some aromatics appear to have amphoteric action, in which they can both stimulate and suppress different parts of the immune system at the same time.

Immunosuppressive aromatics is not an area where we have many human research trials. I'd encourage you to use the *Inflammation Log* found in Appendix A to track your responses to these aromatics. If you're receiving or recovering from chemotherapy, or have recently been ill you may wish to restrict your use of these aromatics.

University of California researchers published their research on mice in *Immunopharmacology* in 1986, finding the constituent of eugenol had a suppressive action on T cells residing in the spleen (splenocytes) when used at low dose, a total inhibition at high dose, and in both doses 'significantly enhanced' natural killer cell activity (Vishteh et al., 1986).

Essential oils rich in eugenol include:
- Clove, bud, stem, and leaf
- Cinnamon, leaf
- Pimento, berry and leaf
- Bay, West Indian
- Holy Basil (Tulsi)

Researchers from the Medical School of Zhejiang University in China published their research on mice in the *Journal of Ethnopharmacology* finding that ginger essential oil suppressed the immune system by inhibiting T cell proliferation and decreasing the overall number of T cells. The authors concluded that the suppressive effect may contribute to ginger's anti-inflammatory activity (Zhou et al., 2006).

List of potential immunosuppressing aromatics:

- Basil, Holy (Tulsi)
- Bay, West Indian
- Cinnamon, leaf
- Clove, bud, stem, and leaf
- Ginger
- Pimento, berry and leaf

From an aromatherapy perspective the anti-inflammatory actions of aromatics is a more widely studied area than the immunosuppressive actions. See chapter 4 *Anti-inflammatory Aromatics* for more aromatics that target suppressing certain immune responses.

4 Anti-inflammatory Aromatics

"Sometimes I need only to stand wherever I am to be blessed." – Mary Oliver

Anti-inflammatory aromatics can have a range of immunosuppressive actions, similar to those discussed in chapter three. For example, the Chinese study on ginger essential oil highlighted an overall decrease in the number of T cells, accounting for an anti-inflammatory activity (Zhou et al., 2006). As with the previous chapter, I recommend using the *Inflammation Log* in Appendix A to track responses to aromatics with a potential anti-inflammatory action, and that those going through or recovering from chemotherapy may wish to limit their use of these types of aromatics.

Another mouse study, undertaken by the Netherland's Department of Infectious Diseases and Immunology in 2009, found one of Oregano's chemical components, carvacrol, activated T cell regulation of inflammation in rheumatoid arthritis (Wieten et al., 2009).

An Italian rat study published in *Pharmacological Research Communications* in 1988 looked at Roman chamomile's anti-inflammatory and sedative properties. The researchers found that the anti-inflammatory effects were still present three hours after dosing (Rossi et al., 1988).

In a 1997 murine study, researchers from the University of Sassari in Italy were interested in whether Clary Sage essential oil's constituents - namely methyl chavicol, linalool, linalyl acetate, and α-terpineol - had an anti-inflammatory action against acute inflammation triggered in rats. They found instead that the essential oil itself had a synergistic effect, working together to produce a stronger anti-inflammatory action than the isolated constituents could offer (Moretti et al., 1997).

Indian researchers from the Amala Cancer Research Centre in Kerala, published their mouse study in the *Indian Journal of Pharmacology* in 2011, finding the essential oil of turmeric reduced both acute and chronic inflammation (Liju et al., 2011).

Boswellia Resin

The Boswellia species, perhaps better known as Frankincense, is a group of 25 different species of trees indigenous to Ethiopia, Somalia, Saudi Arabia, Yemen, and Oman (Koeppen 2015). While the linalool, 1-octanol, and α-pinene found in the essential oil have topical anti-inflammatory properties (Li et al., 2016), the real sweet spot with this botanical isn't found in appreciable numbers in the essential oil. The Boswellia species has more than 12 different boswellic acids, including the promising 11-Keto-β-Boswellic acid, and the Acetyl-11-keto-β-Boswellic acid. Boswellic acids, or BAs for short, decrease the production of proinflammatory cytokines which can show up in chronic inflammatory conditions in the cartilage, insulin producing cells, bronchial, intestines, and other tissues (Ammon 2016).

I've selected a handful of studies that look at different types of chronic inflammation and the benefits of standardized extracts of Boswellia tree resins:

- **Asthma** – 40 patient study showed 70% had improvements taking Boswellia serrata resin for 6 weeks (Gupta et al., 1998).

- **Colitis** – 30 patient study showed 80% remission taking Boswellia serrata for 6 weeks for ulcerative colitis (Gupta et al., 2001); 31 patient study showed higher remission in those taking Boswellia serrata resin for 6 weeks for collagenous colitis (Madisch et al., 2007).

- **Crohn's Disease** – 102 patient study found 8 weeks of Boswellia serrata resin dosing to work similarly to mesalazine (mesalamine) (Gerhardt et al., 2001).

- **Multiple Sclerosis** – 38 patient study for an 8 month trial using standardized frankincense resin extract for 8 months showed positive clinical outcomes, the resin did not affect lymphocyte count (Stürner et al., 2017).

- **Osteoarthritis** – 90 patient study showed improvement in pain scale with an Ayurvedic formula of Ashwaganda (*Withania somnifera*) , Boswellia serrrata, Ginger (*Zingiber officinale*), and Turmeric (*Curcumin longa*) (Chopra et al., 2004); 49 patient study showed improvements with shorter duration of tenderness, more walking time, and less joint swelling taking Boswellia carteri resin and turmeric for 90 days (Badria et al., 2002); 66 patient study showed slow onset of action followed by persistent effects a month following the 32 week study taking Boswellia serrata resin (Sontakke et al., 2007).

List of potential anti-inflammatory aromatics:

- Bergamot
- Blue Mallee
- Boswellia resin
- Cajuput

- Cardamom
- Chamomile, Roman
- Clary Sage
- Coriander
- Eucalyptus citriodora
- Eucalyptus globulus
- Eucalyptus smithii
- Geranium
- Ho Leaf ct cineole
- Lavandin, super
- Lavender
- Niaouli ct cineole
- Oregano
- Palmarosa
- Petitgrain, bigarade
- Rosalina
- Rosemary ct cineole
- Thyme ct linalool
- Turmeric

Join me in part two to apply this foundation of potential immune modulating aromatics to your wellness plan.

PART II: AROMATIC THERAPIES IN PRACTICE

5 The Immune-Mind Connection

"There are days I drop words of comfort on myself like falling leaves and remember that it is enough to be taken care of by my self." – Brian Andreas

You may not be surprised to hear that emotions have an impact on the immune system. If you've ever been under pressure to work on a deadline and got a head cold or UTI as soon as you came up for breath, you know just what I'm talking about!

In this chapter we'll explore how grief, childhood trauma, and chronic stress influence immunity. As an aromatherapist I love seeing this kind of research because it helps us to better understand how we got sick in the first place and gives us tools to support the healing process. It's that bridge - modern science paired with the healing art of aromatic therapies - that gives us a whole-person approach to wellness.

Let's take a closer look at some of the research behind the immune-mind connection.

Psychoneuroimmunology

Researchers have been studying what is known as *psychoneuroimmunology* (or PNI) for several decades, helping us to better understand the immune-mind connection. PNI is the study of how emotions influence immunity and how immunity influences emotions via the autonomic nervous system (Ziemssen et al., 2007).

Stress, for example, will trigger the stress system to shift into what is known as the "fight or flight" response. This is controlled by one branch of the autonomic nervous system, the sympathetic nervous system (SNS). The SNS releases norepinephrine hormone to trigger an increase in heart rate, dilate blood vessels in the arms and legs, pause digestion, and release glucose energy into the bloodstream. The SNS also suppresses immunity, which is of particular concern for those of us relying on the immune system to manage inflammation. In reverse, when the immune system is fighting infection, it can actually trigger a release of stress hormones, which causes mood and cognition issues as well as further suppresses the immune response. The suppression of the immune system through the stress system isn't a uniform action though; it can cause short-term and long-term changes, and trigger exaggerated immune and inflammation reactions (Dhabhar 2009; Elenkov 1999).

Psychoneuroimmunology is thought to be a contributing factor in:
- Chronic fatigue syndrome - Glaser et al., 1998.
- Depression - Dantzer et al., 2008.
- Immune changes in children - Marin et al., 2009.
- Some types of cancer - Kiecolt-Glaser et al., 2002.
- Pregnancy & postpartum mental health disorders - Sherer et al., 2017.
- Rheumatoid arthritis - Irwin et al., 2002.

Those who are more vulnerable to immune challenges may find psychoneuroimmunology helps explain why their autoimmune or inflammatory conditions become exacerbated, recur after a period of remission, or markedly progress during and following periods of strong emotions.

Adverse Childhood Experiences

Another area of research looks at the impact that childhood emotional trauma has on the immature immune system (Buranen 2013). Adverse childhood experiences, or ACEs for short, can include emotional or physical neglect, emotional or physical abuse, bullying, the death of a loved one, parents separating or divorcing, incarceration of a loved one, food insecurity, or a loved one with a mental illness. In 2009, researchers from the National Center for Disease Prevention and Health Promotion found that adults who had experienced traumatic childhood stressors had an increased likelihood of being hospitalized with a diagnosed autoimmune condition decades into adulthood (Dube et Al., 2009).

When we combine our knowledge of the impacts emotional stressors have on the adult immune system it is easier to understand how this can be magnified in the case of an underdeveloped immune system in a child's body.

Grief

In 1983, doctors from Mount Sinai Hospital in New York published a study in the Journal of the American Medical Association about the increased risk of illness (morbidity) and death (mortality) following the death of a spouse to breast cancer. The study found these widowers experienced a suppressed immunity for up to 14 months following the death of their loved one (Schleifer et al., 1983).

A more recent study, published in 2003 in the journal Psychiatry Research, looked at the immune, endocrine, and psychological responses to patients following *"unpredictable acute emotional stress (e.g. sudden death of a loved one)."* They found those who were grieving were profoundly stressed 10 days after the event. At the 40 day follow-up their natural killer (NK) cells were *markedly reduced*, and while some were faring better - emotionally speaking - at the six-month follow-up, their immune systems were still impacted all those months later (Gerra et al., 2003).

My paternal grandmother passed away in early 2017 after a brief illness. My wellness plan took shape the day after her death when I started meditating with the smartphone app *Insight Timer*, in particular the comforting Irish accent of Tony Brady in his recording, *Support in a Time of Bereavement*. My meditations were anchored with aromatics, from frankincense resin burning on the bamboo charcoal, a splash of neroli hydrosol in a glass of water, or an aromastick of my favorite supportive essential oils including Cypress, Himalayan Cedarwood, and a hint of Rose. Aromatics during bereavement give us an opportunity to gently support the suppressed immune response using a backdoor – the mind-immune connection of psychoneuroimmunology.

Aromatics and Psychoneuroimmunology

Since psychoneuroimmunology is a two-way street, we can use key aromatics to shift the nervous system from a "fight or flight" autonomic response to a "rest and digest" autonomic response, better known as the parasympathetic nervous system (PSNS). Our bodies rely on the ability to move into the parasympathetic nervous system throughout the day to rest, assess energy needs, and maintain homeostasis in the endocrine, digestive, and cardiovascular systems.

A handful of years ago I ran across a theory by psychology researcher, Ernest Rossi. The theory divided the 24-hour body clock, known as the *circadian rhythm*, into a shorter clock that allowed for 90-120 minutes of mental and physical activity followed by 15-20 minutes of rest. These shorter body cycles are known as ultradian rhythms, and Rossi co-wrote about his theory in the 1991 book *The Twenty Minute Break: Reduce Stress, Maximize Performance, Improve Health and Emotional Well-Being Using the New Science of Ultradian Rhythms*.

I decided to combine Rossi's theory and add in a limbic brain tie-in with aromatics to gently nudge the body back into the PSNS during these 20 minute breaks. To anchor the break, and clearly delineate "work" time from "rest/break" time, I would use an aromastick with a blend of aromatic volatiles I found pleasant but neither stimulating nor sedating. Every couple of hours I would grab my aromastick, take a deep inhalation from it from both nostrils, and take a break for 15-20 minutes, then return to what I was doing previously. After a few days I found I was emotionally calmer, didn't react to stressors with the same intensity as previously, and my sleep cycles were more harmonious. That's when I decided to start having my clients that were struggling with time management, premenstrual syndrome, insomnia, chronic stress, depression, anxiety, and grief start using this ultradian rhythm aromastick theory. The feedback was fantastic, and I was pleased to have the opportunity to share my approach with colleagues at the Alliance of

International Aromatherapists' 2015 conference in Denver, Colorado in my talk *Holistic Support for Mental Wellness: Practical Tips for Aromatherapists.* See Chapter Ten for a template of an *Ultradian Rhythm Aromastick* formulation.

Combining Aromatics with Other Mind-Body Therapies

If you'd like to take it a step further, I'd recommend pairing your aromastick or another aromatic intervention with one or more of the following therapies:

- Meditation and Yoga Nidra – yoga studios frequently host meditation classes; I also really like the Insight Timer smartphone app for guided meditation.
- Yoga – think gentle, restorative yoga.
- Talk therapy – works well when combined with cognitive behavioral therapy to reduce dysfunctional psychosomatic patterns and boost happiness. Rachel Hershenberg's 2017 book *Activating Happiness: A Jump-Start Guide to Overcoming Low Motivation, Depression, or Just Feeling Stuck* is a good resource for CBT work on your own terms.
- Acupuncture – you might even get lucky and have a practitioner who has trained with Peter Holmes in aroma acupoint therapy, which is a beautiful synergy of these two modalities!
- Reflexology – I'm biased as a board certified practitioner of reflexology for the past fourteen years, but we're not joking when we say an hour of reflexology is like getting a four-hour power nap. I've yet to find a modality that induces relaxation as effectively as a session with a qualified reflexologist. Check with your local professional reflexology association for a referral near you.

Direct inhalation of essential oils is our quickest route to the limbic portion of the brain, where the autonomic nervous system is controlled. We can use aromatics that elicit calm in the face of stress, shifting us from a place of a "fight or flight" sympathetic nervous (SNS) state to the "rest and digest" parasympathetic nervous (PSNS) state. In my practice I routinely use aromasticks for clients with PTSD, acute and chronic emotional trauma, generalized anxiety disorder, autoimmune and inflammatory conditions, and for other types of mood support and regulation.

6 Aromatic Therapies and Immune Stimulation

"A child who is protected from all controversial ideas is as vulnerable as a child who is protected from every germ. The infection, when it comes - and it will come - may overwhelm the system, be it the immune system or the belief system."
- Jane Smiley

Constantly diffusing "germ fighting" essential oils and otherwise stimulating the immune system all cold and flu season is not a holistic approach to wellness. Every holistic system I have studied, Ancient Greek Medicine, Traditional Chinese Medicine, Ayurveda, Curanderismo (latin folk healing), Ancient Iranian/Pakistani Medicine (Tibb-e-Unani), and Western Herbal Medicine, focuses on supporting the terrain for cold and flu prevention and wellness. What are the far-reaching implications of having the immune system stimulated all season long? What about immunostimulation in the underdeveloped immune systems of children? What are we losing if a child is not fully exercising their immunity?

Caring for the terrain, the body, is fundamental to prevention and wellness in holistic medicine. Key areas of terrain support include sleep hygiene, hydration, exercise, stress management, and maintaining a healthy integumentary system. Let's explore these fundamental elements of wellness and how aromatics can play a role.

Insomnia as a Proinflammatory

Sleep and immunity have a reciprocal relationship (Bryant et al., 2004). Sleep deprivation can lead to an increase in inflammatory markers and an increased risk of compromised immunity. There is an increased risk of developing sleep disorders like insomnia, restless leg syndrome, and obstructive sleep apnea with a dysregulated immune system in cases like HIV, multiple sclerosis, and Lyme disease, (Gamaldo et al., 2012). Innate immunity is altered in those who have shift work schedules, jet lag, and circadian rhythm disorders (Castanon-Cervantes et al., 2010).

We can employ sedative and relaxant essential oils to support healthy sleep hygiene during periods of insomnia (Lillehei et al., 2014). I like to combine aromatics like Sweet Marjoram, Lavender, Neroli, or West Australian Sandalwood with guided meditation, like Yoga Nidra to support sleep hygiene. Try putting a drop of Sweet Marjoram on a tissue, tuck it inside the pillow case, and queue up your meditation track.

Dehydration and Innate Immunity

Dehydration not only stresses the integrity of the skin and mucous membranes - our first line of defense against pathogens - but it can cause the antimicrobial proteins in the mucosal tissues to decrease leaving us more vulnerable to the invasion of microbes (Fortes et al., 2012).

In my 2017 book, *Aromatic Waters*, I give a number of recipes on using hydrosols to enhance the flavor and therapeutics of beverages. For those with a dysregulated or underactive thirst reflex a teaspoon or two of cinnamon, geranium, or rose hydrosol to a pitcher of filtered water can be a nice incentive to consume more liquids during the day. Antioxidant rich berries and fruit can be blended into water to enhance flavor and therapeutics as well. Technology may be helpful; I frequently recommend my clients download a smartphone app that will remind them to hydrate at intervals during the day.

Vitamin D's Role in Immune Wellness

Micronutrient deficiency can impact immune response in a number of ways. Take vitamin D_3, an immunosuppressive hormone with the ability to suppress the development of various autoimmune diseases (Cantorna et al., 2004). It is also considered a beneficial tool to prevent respiratory infections during cold and flu season (Martineau et al., 2017).

Sedentary Lifestyle and the Immune System

Too much exercise can suppress immune function and is linked to upper respiratory tract infections (Smith et al., 2003). As well, a sedentary lifestyle appears to lead to pro-inflammatory immune responses and is thought to be the culprit behind a number of lifestyle diseases, like diabetes (Kolb et al., 2010).

I've used aromatic botanicals in a number of client wellness plans to help incentivize exercise, or loving movement of the body. How? If one has a negative association with exercise it makes it hard to find that motivation to go to the gym. In my 2011 research study for my clinical aromatherapy training, I asked the question *"Can the essential oil Cupressus sempervirens compare to commercial antiperspirant deodorants for under arm odor and moisture control?"* I wanted to find out if Cypress essential oil would be a good alternative to commercial deodorants that employ aluminum and is contraindicated for clients with breast cancer. My volunteers used a Cypress formulation in one axilla (armpit) and their regular antiperspirant deodorant in the other axilla. While my small pool of eleven volunteers found they got about eight hours of coverage out of the Cypress before they had to reapply, several surprised me telling me they enjoyed their workouts in the gym more with the Cypress than they had previously. Since then I've used Cypress as a key aromatic in inhaled aromatic formulas for clients to take a deep whiff of just before hitting the treadmill, spinning class, or yoga flow class, and it works really well. Try adding Cypress to another favorite aromatic that is invigorating and refreshing (think peppermint, lemon, and eucalyptus), and put it either in an aromastick you carry in your pocket to the gym or on a diffuser bracelet or necklace for discreet inhalation.

Prefer outdoor activities instead? Try the Japanese concept of *Shinrin-yoku*, or forest bathing. Researchers at the Japanese public health department and forestry institute have found the benefits of walking in the forest are more beneficial than a walk through a bustling city setting (Li et al., 2011). Forest bathing gives us a welcome dose of nature's own aromatherapy through the release of aromatic constituents. Nothing beats going right to the source!

In 2008, Colorado researchers published a literature review in *Trends in Immunology* recommending the therapeutic value of a common bacteria found in soil, *Mycobacterium vaccae* (Rook et Al., 2008). They noted that M. vaccae could induce an immune regulatory response, showing promising results for persons with anxiety or depression paired with a chronic inflammatory conditions. I think it makes a good case for spending time gardening and playing in the soil, and have found that in the handful of years I've been unable to garden due to apartment life, my mood and immunity took a hit. These days, you'll find me spending time digging in the dirt a few times a week in my apothecary garden year-round.

Aromatics and Skin Hygiene

The skin is part of our innate defense system against microbes and is home to a diverse range of microorganisms (Grice et al., 2009). If we lose that diversity of the skin microbiota we're more susceptible to atopic dermatitis, acne vulgaris, plaque psoriasis, and poor wound healing (Kong et al., 2012). In cases where single strain organisms are causing skin disorders, aromatic massage could be used to help modulate the root microbiome (Donoyama et al., 2005, 2006). Many essential oils and CO_2 extracts have antimicrobial actions and can be used to restore lost harmony to the skin. When I wish to employ an aromatic massage oil in a professional massage I ask my practitioner about known allergens, and scent preferences. Then I formulate a body oil at 2-3%, see Appendix B for a dilution chart, and bring it with me to my next massage. In the case of infectious skin conditions - Athlete's foot fungus, staphylococcal infections like MRSA or cellulitis - I choose self-massage in the Ayurvedic tradition to avoid infecting my practitioner. You'll find a recipe for Aromatic Self-Massage in Chapter Ten.

Stress Reduction

We previously explored the impact of the stress system on the immune system in the Immune-Mind Connection chapter, though it bears repeating that aromatics can be a great tool for stress reduction (Hwang 2006). In fact, if you're looking to address chronic inflammation and prevent disease, stress reduction has the potential to help you reach those goals (O'Byrne et al., 2001; Dalgleish et al., 2002).

7 Aromatic Therapies and Cancer

"I know that if odour were visible, as colour is, I'd see the summer garden in rainbow clouds" – Robert Bridges

Some aromatics have the potential to be chemopreventive, which means they may be able to interrupt the process of normal cells transforming into cancer cells, known as carcinogenesis. We can harness these aromatics as part of a cancer prevention wellness plan that addresses reducing lifestyle risk factors, encouraging homeostasis in multiple systems and promoting overall health.

Western medicine approaches cancer treatment with chemotherapeutic drugs, radiation, surgical removal of tumors, and immunotherapy interventions. Chemotherapy targets cells that divide quickly, a trait of cancer cells as well as lymphocytes. Aromatics that would stimulate lymphocyte production could make the chemo less effective, while aromatics that suppress lymphocyte production could potentiate the chemo to a greater degree than the oncology team was prepared for. During chemo, precautions are taken to reduce exposure of microbes while the immune system is vulnerable, including thorough washing of fresh produce and avoiding handling and eating raw or undercooked foods. Other aromatics that would be prudent to avoid would be those that use the same pathways of metabolism through the liver that a medication does and those that thin the blood.

Following chemotherapy, the road to recovery can be lengthy for some types of cancer. Take breast cancer for example, repopulation of lymphocytes following chemo for this cancer can take up to nine months (Verma et al., 2016). Aromatics that may stimulate lymphocyte production and the immune system, like the ones mentioned in chapter 2, have the potential to reduce recovery periods.

Aromatics as Part of a Cancer Prevention Wellness Plan

"Prevention is better than cure." - Desiderius Erasmus

When we look at the literature exploring lifestyle risk factors for cancer many signs point at chronic stress and our Western culture of "busyness." The University of Sydney did a literature review of 103 cohort studies to determine which lifestyle risk factors were at play with colorectal cancer. The researchers found that alcohol consumption, smoking, diabetes, obesity, and high meat intakes were associated with increased risk of colorectal cancer (Huxley et al., 2009). Many of our vices, like nicotine and alcohol, are stress-coping tools for the harried adult. Have you ever noticed that those amongst us who take regular breaks from work and actually mentally check-out for their 15-minute break, are nicotine users? How many of us find it natural to jump-start the day with caffeine and wind-down with alcohol? These are stress coping tools, as poor for our health as they are, and we've grown accustomed to them.

What if we harnessed aromatic therapies to decrease lifestyle risk factors by gently nudging the individual towards improved wellness? Instead of reaching for nicotine every 90 minutes we used an aromastick? Let's look at some key areas where we could employ aromatics in a cancer preventative lifestyle.

Sleep as a Chemopreventive

In chapter six we looked at the proinflammatory relationship of dysregulated sleep cycles with the body. Insomnia puts us at an increased risk of prostate (Sigurdardottir et al., 2013), colorectal (Thompson et al., 2011), and breast cancer (Thompson et al., 2012). The production of the hormone melatonin by the pineal gland enhances immune function, facilitates sleep, and inhibits the development and growth of cancer (Blask 2009).

In an Aromatic Wellness Plan for Cancer Prevention we could use sedative and relaxant essential oils to support healthy sleep hygiene during periods of insomnia (Lillehei et al., 2014).

Hydration as a Chemopreventive

Research shows water intake reduces colon cancer risk for both men and women (Shannon 1996), and bladder cancer risk for men (Michaud 1999). For some of us, staying hydrated is second-nature and doesn't require much consideration or planning. That's not the case with all of us though, so if you're in the group of us who need some planning and regular reminders this a lifestyle factor you can start working on.

The National Academy of Medicine, formerly the Institute of Medicine, recommends a daily fluid intake of 91 ounces for women and 125 ounces for men who have more sedentary jobs or lifestyles, are in good health, and live in a temperate climate, places that have four major seasons (Institute of Medicine 2005). About 20% of our fluid intake comes from food sources like fresh fruits and vegetables, soups, even a morning cup of black tea or coffee.

Hydration needs increase for those who are exposed to high temperatures for prolonged periods of time, basically anyone who spends a good chunk of their day outdoors in hot summers, and those who have more strenuous lifestyles either through exercise or occupations that require manual labor tasks most of the time.

One of the easier ways to measure additional water intake needs is to actually measure water loss:

- Prior to the activity get on the scale and take a base weight.
- Track water intake while you're mowing the lawn, working out at the gym, or other physical activities.
- Towel-off any sweat, and wearing the same items you were wearing with the first weigh-in, reweigh yourself.
- Calculate the overall weight loss from the activity.
- Then add the water you consumed during the activity (water weighs 0.065 pounds per ounce so an 8 ounce glass of water would weigh 0.52 pounds).

Hydrosols, the water distillate obtained in the process of distillation, have helped a number of my clients increase and maintain their water intake. In my 2017 book *Aromatic Waters: Therapeutic, Cosmetic, and Culinary Hydrosol Applications*, I give a number of recipes on using hydrosols to enhance the flavor and therapeutics of beverages.

Technology is a great tool to stay mindful of water intake throughout the day. I recommend to clients that are struggling with hydration getting a smartphone app like *Waterlogged, Daily Water*, or *Hydro Coach*.

Plan to Eat More Spices

Aromatic spices have chemopreventive properties (Lai et al., 2004) and can be used in cooking on a daily basis. Being a fan of food-as-medicine, which posits food as the most powerful drug on the planet with the capacity to be beneficial or harmful, I think we should all be eating more spices. Antioxidant-rich spices like ginger (*Zingiber officinale*) have the potential to affect the proliferation and progression of cancer by preventing free radical formation and damage, reducing inflammation, and stimulating programmed cell death - apoptosis (Lamp et al., 2003). Turmeric's powerful constituent curcumin has been found to be more potent at free radical scavenging than vitamin E (Zhao et al., 1989), and has been studied for a variety of cancers including its in vitro inhibition of breast cancer cells (Bachmeier et al., 2007).

If you're looking for inspiration on stocking and using aromatic spices in the kitchen I recommend the following books: *Spices that Heal* by Tieroana Low Dog, MD (Medicine Lodge Ranch); Arun Kapil's *Fresh Spice: Vibrant Recipes for Bringing Flavour, Depth and Colour to Home Cooking* (Pavilion 2014); and Rosalee de la Forêt's *Alchemy of Herbs: Transform Everyday Ingredients into Foods and Remedies That Heal* (Hay House 2017). I've included a recipe for the Ayurvedic dish *Kitchari* in chapter ten to jump-start cooking your way through the spice cabinet.

Skin Cancer Prevention

One in five Americans will be diagnosed with skin cancer by the age of 70 (Stern 2010). Ultraviolet radiation mutates DNA, thus contributing to the initiation phase of carcinogenesis (Stratton et al 2006). The immune system responds to UV radiation by sending proinflammatory cytokines to the dermal layer (Strickland et al., 1997). In my Apothecary Session class titled *Aromatic Beauty Care,* I teach students how to harness anti-inflammatory aromatics and lipids as well as antioxidant botanical extracts for daily skincare products. We formulate to protect against the free radical damage of ultraviolet radiation using ingredients like polyphenol-rich green tea (*Camellia sinensis*) and the antioxidant and anti-inflammatory rich punicic acid from pomegranate seed oil.

Here's a formula from my 2017 book *Aromatic Waters: Therapeutic, Cosmetic, and Culinary Hydrosol Applications:*

Frankincense Gel Serum

60 mls Frankincense hydrosol
650 mg Xanthan or Sclerotium gum
600 mg glucanolactone and sodium benzoate

In a medium-sized bowl, gently heat the hydrosol until it is lukewarm. Add the powdered gum and the GSB preservative and whisk until smooth. Use a cosmetic brush, cotton pad, or sponge to apply a thin coat to the face, paying extra attention to areas that need more hydration.

Aromatic Breast Wellness

Pomegranate seed oil is one of my favorite lipids to use in a breast massage oil formulation. It is rich in punicic acid, a long-chain polyunsaturated fatty acid which has shown *in vitro* activity inhibiting breast cancer cell growth (Grossman et al., 2010). I combine it here with anti-inflammatory essential oils of Turmeric and Frankincense, and limonene-rich citrus essential oils. Robert Tisserand has written an insightful article on the use of *Citrus Oils and Breast Health* on his website tisserandinstitute.org that I highly recommend reading.

5 mls Pomegranate Seed Oil
15 mls Sweet Almond Oil
2 drops Turmeric essential oil
3 drops Boswellia sacra essential oil
10 drops Lemon essential oil

Combine lipid oils and essential oils in a 1 ounce dropper bottle, shake well to combine, massage 10-15 drops into breasts using sweeping motions up towards the armpit. Breastfeeding women should avoid applications to the nipple and areola.

Immunomodulatory Aromatics for Cancer Recovery

Aromatics that stimulate and amplify the immune system, like the ones mentioned in chapter two, may reduce recovery time following chemotherapy. Talk with your oncologist about the best time to start aromatherapy or herbal supplements like *Cordyceps sinensis*. A number of my clients have received the green light shortly after the last round of chemo.

I would also recommend exploring the Ultradian Rhythm Aromastick and the Aromatic Self-Massage recipes found in chapter ten.

8 Aromatic Therapies and Autoimmune Conditions

"The Herbs ought to be distilled when they are in their greatest vigor, and so ought the Flowers also." - Nicholas Culpeper

In autoimmune conditions, the immune system destroys normal tissue instead of antigens. One area of research has looked at the impact on autoimmune and chronic inflammatory conditions when natural killer T cells are in short supply or have functional deficiencies (Fogel et al., 2013).

Those who are more vulnerable to immune challenges may find psychoneuroimmunology, discussed in chapter five, helps explain why their autoimmune or inflammatory conditions become exacerbated, recur after a period of remission, or markedly progress during and following periods of strong emotions.

As discussed in previous chapters, aromatics to support chronic inflammation and a dysregulated immune system could include focus work on:

- Sleep Hygiene
- Hydration
- Stress Reduction
- Combining Aromatics with Other Mind-Body Therapies

Additional tools in the remainder of this book for autoimmunity include chapter nine covering chronic inflammation, chapter ten's aromatic recipes, and the Inflammation Log found in Appendix A. Use the log to help you determine whether your aromatic intervention(s) are reducing symptoms, assisting with remission, potentially triggering a flare, relapse, or worsening of symptoms. Share these results with your wellness team – your aromatherapist, rheumatologist, osteopath, functional medicine physician, et cetera.

9 Aromatic Therapies and Chronic Inflammation

"Flowers always make people better, happier, and more helpful; they are sunshine, food and medicine for the soul." - Luther Burbank

We recognize inflammation as pain, swelling, heat, and tissue redness; and it is the body's response to injury, irritant, or invasion by an infectious agent (Stevens et al., 2016). Inflammation is an immune-guided response that sends a type of white blood cells, called neutrophils, to the affected area. These respond to an infection by ingesting the pathogen and releasing enzymes that kill that pathogen. Neutrophils in wound healing assist in breaking down the injured tissue so the lymphocytes can come in and help remove it and speed up the healing process.

Chronic inflammation involves constant immune stimulation. It can look like poor concentration, fatigue, bloating, muscle and joint pain, or a general feeling of being unwell. It can contribute to inflammatory bowel disease (IBD), infertility, rheumatoid arthritis, chronic fatigue syndrome, asthma, periodontitis, sinusitis, some cancers, over a hundred autoimmune conditions, and more. Functional medicine physicians like Susan Blum, author of the 2013 book "The Immune System Recovery Plan: A Doctor's 4-step Program to Treat Autoimmune Disease," talk about triggers that set off chronic inflammation. These triggers can include food sensitivities, environmental toxins, and chronic stress.

According to the Harvard Women's Health Watch (2014), foods that contribute to inflammation include refined carbohydrates, fried foods, sugar-sweetened beverages, red meat, processed meat, margarine, shortening, and lard.

As discussed in previous chapters, aromatics to support chronic inflammation and a dysregulated immune system could include focus work on:
- Sleep Hygiene
- Hydration
- Stress Reduction

- Combining Aromatics with Other Mind-Body Therapies

You'll find aromatic recipes in the next chapter that can be customized to include anti-inflammatory aromatics previously discussed in Part One.

10 Aromatic Recipes

"Mother Earth's medicine chest is full of healing herbs of incomparable worth."
- Robin Rose Bennet

While it is hard to produce one-size-fits-all recipes for autoimmunity, cancer prevention, and chronic inflammation, I've included some of my favorites here. You'll notice that these focus on enhancing wellness through gentle lifestyle modifications. I encourage you to reference the lists found in Part One of this book to create a customized aromatherapy experience. The appendix features two charts I think you'll find useful - the first to track symptoms and the second to give you some dosing guidelines that represent the industry's best practices.

Aromatic Self-Massage

Oil massage, known as *abhyanga*, has been a part of Ayurveda for thousands of years (Pole 2006). It is one of the central features of a daily wellness regimen and a practice I recommend to many of my clients. A small amount of warmed oil - like sesame, jojoba, or avocado - is massaged into the skin prior to the morning shower. If I have the time in my morning routine, I start with *garshana* (dry-brushing). *Garshana* gently massages the skin with a natural bristle brush, starting at the feet and moving upwards towards the heart.

Abyhanga nourishes the skin, soothes the nervous system, promotes good digestion, and helps the immune system remove waste material by circulating the lymph. Start at the feet, move up the legs, and then switch to the hands and arms. Massage the belly and lower back, the chest, shoulders, neck, scalp. Finish with the face.

When I make my 'Aby' massage oil I use the following template:
- 6 drops of a favorite tree oil (e.g. cypress, sandalwood, juniper, cedarwood)
- 4 drops of a favorite floral (e.g. geranium, rose, jasmine absolute)
- 2 drops of a favorite citrus (e.g. grapefruit, red or green mandarin, sweet orange) or petitgrain
- and 1 drop of either a warming essential oil (e.g. ginger, cardamom,

coriander) if you've got a cool constitution

Based on your wellness goals, you may wish to select from aromatics that will potentially reduce inflammation or one of the other immunemodulatory actions described in Part One. Use this template as a guideline and mix or match the aromatics that will be the most effective for your needs and constitution.

'Aby' Massage Oil - a 2.5% Dilution

30 mls or 1 ounce Sesame, Jojoba, or Avocado Oil
15 drops essential oils

In a one ounce glass dropper bottle, add your selected essential oils and lipid oil. Gently shake to combine. Use 5-10 drops at a time, rubbing between the palms of your hands and then massaging into the body using the instructions above.

Since you will be jumping in the shower or bath following the massage, the heat and water will help drive the aromatics deeper into your tissues. Note that you're not greasing up here! In the summer months I use 5-10 mls, or 1-2 teaspoons, in the dry autumn and winter I use 10-30mls.

Kitchari

I frequently recommend a porridge-like Indian dish known as Kitchari to my clients as a way to introduce more aromatic spices into their diet and gently reset the gastrointestinal system, as part of a seasonal cleanse. Kitchari is traditionally serves as baby's introduction to solid foods, for those recovering from illness, and for those on a physical or spiritual cleanse. You could enjoy this dish as an occasional meal or in a cleanse format eat it for each meal for three days.

2 cups white basmati rice
1 cup split yellow mung dahl beans
2 teaspoons clarified butter (ghee)
3-5 whole cardamom pods
½-1 inch fresh minced ginger root (or 1-2 teaspoons powdered)
1 teaspoon coriander seed
1 teaspoon cumin seed
¼-1 teaspoon turmeric powder
1-2 teaspoons peppercorn
1 cinnamon or cassia stick
1 teaspoon black or yellow mustard seeds
½ teaspoon fenugreek seeds
2-3 cloves
3 bay leaves
½ teaspoon salt

7-10 cups water (6 cups if using pressure cooker)

Stovetop instructions: add rice and beans to a large pot and bring to a boil. Reduce heat, cover, and simmer until rice and beans are tender. In a separate pan, sauté spices and ghee on medium heat until fragrant. Add to rice and beans. Just before serving add chopped, fresh cilantro, or parsley.

If rice is problematic, tapioca starch - which is made from cassava root - can be used instead. Mung dahl is a low FODMAP bean but could be replaced with quinoa or millet if it isn't well tolerated. You'll find kitchari is quite versatile and can be rolled up in a whole grain or cassava tortilla, served on a bed of spring greens, or in a broth as a soup.

Ultradian Rhythm Aromastick

My favorite form of direct inhalation is using a device known as an aromastick. Aromasticks are available in plastic or metal housing and have a wick to hold drops of essential oils, absolutes, and CO2 extracts. You hold the aromastick up to the nose, inhale deeply in one nostril, remove, breath regularly for a few breaths, then repeat on the opposite nostril.

Choose 3 of the following aromatics:
- Calming & Cooling: Geranium, Jasmine, Mandarin (Red or Green), Neroli, Rose
- Centering: Black Spruce, Cypress, Scot's Pine, Cedarwood (Atlas or Himalayan), Juniper Berry, Western Australian Sandalwood, Frankincense
- Uplifting: Bergamot, Lemongrass, Sweet Orange

Take out the cotton wick of your aromastick, put it in a shallow dish and add 12-18 drops of the aromatics you've chosen. Return the wick to the inner housing, push the cap in, twist on the outer housing, and it is ready to ride around in your pocket with you all day. Use the timer on your smartphone to gently buzz or chime at you every two hours for your aroma break.

11 Working with an Aromatherapist

"Some people believe aromatherapy means just inhalation. Others believe aromatherapy means aromatherapy massage. Physicians in France define aromatherapy to mean the inclusion of essential oils via oral, rectal, and vaginal routes. Clearly, different levels of types of training are required and need to be relevant to the student."
- Jane Buckle, Clinical Aromatherapy: Essential Oils in Healthcare

Here in the United States aromatherapy is a self-governing healing arts modality, and our education guidelines come from organizations like the Alliance of International Aromatherapists (AIA), the National Association for Holistic Aromatherapy (NAHA), and the Aromatherapy Registration Council (ARC). Those who market themselves as an aromatherapist are expected to meet these national education guidelines, though there is no law requiring them to do so. Depending on what type of aromatherapy services and the depth of consultation you are looking for you may wish to choose amongst the most common tiers of education:

1. Entry-level aromatherapist - someone who has had a foundation course in aromatherapy of about 100 hours, including basic anatomy and physiology, and a working knowledge of about 20 essential oils.

2. Certified or professional aromatherapist - in addition to a foundations course in aromatherapy, this person should have deeper training in a handful of health conditions, have a working knowledge of about 40 essential oils, and have some consultation skills. This is usually an additional 100 hours for a total of 200 hours.

3. Advanced level - in addition to the other two levels, this person should have a solid understanding of pathologies, a deeper training in anatomy and physiology, and a working knowledge of about 50 essential oils. Clinical aromatherapists generally fall into this category and have received specialized training specific to clinical practice. This is usually an additional 100-200 hours for a total of 300-400 hours.

4. Advanced clinical aromatherapy - through continuing education the practitioner is trained in internal dose forms including oral, rectal, vaginal, buccal, and nebulized doses. This advanced training may be called Aromatic Medicine, and is sometimes called by the term French Aromatherapy. This is

usually a 100-500 hour program and is usually only taught to those who have been in practice for several years at an advanced levels. Someone with this level of training usually has a minimum of 600 hours of formal education in the aromatic therapies but could be upwards of 900-1,500 hours dependent on the other continuing education the practitioner has done.

Consulting with an aromatherapist gives you a unique opportunity to discuss your wellness goals, and health history and receive a customized treatment plan in return. Every aromatic has dosing guidelines, condition interactions, medication interactions, and special considerations for age and constitution. Your aromatherapist will carefully take these into consideration when preparing a wellness plan for you.

To find an aromatherapist near you, I recommend contacting your local aromatherapy association for a referral. I've included a list of aromatherapy associations in the Resources in Appendix C.

Epilogue

"Do you know what you are? You are a manuscript of a divine letter. You are a mirror reflecting a noble face. This universe is not outside of you. Look inside yourself; everything that you want, you are already that." - Rumi

In Part One we looked at research from the scientific community which can help us narrow down which aromatics may become cherished aromatic allies. Part Two had us exploring the fascinating mind-immune connection and other ways to integrate these botanicals into customized wellness plans.

As we've explored in this book, aromatherapy is a holistic modality that can safely and gently nudge a dysregulated immune system towards homeostasis. It can also play a role in the prevention of immune dysregulation as part of a healthy lifestyle to defend against cancer, autoimmunity, and chronic inflammation. One of the many reasons I love aromatherapy is how accessible it is for self-care to enhance wellbeing.

For aromatherapy to remain safe and effective for individuals with dysregulated immune systems we need to understand the potential advantages and disadvantages of the individual aromatics' use. My hope is that this volume will assist you in making informed decisions about how you use aromatic therapies to reach your equilibrium goals. Wishing you and yours abundant health!

Appendix A: Inflammation Log

1. Starting Level of Pain

0	1	2	3	4	5	6	7	8	9	10

No Pain   Moderate   Extreme Pain

2. Location(s) and Intensity of Pain

Head	Neck	Back	Shoulder	Arm	Glute	Hip	Leg
□None □Mild □Moderate □Severe	□None □Mild □Moderate □Severe	□None □Mild □Moderate □Severe	□None □Mild □Moderate □Severe	□None □Mild □Moderate □Severe	□None □Mild □Moderate □Severe	□None □Mild □Moderate □Severe	□None □Mild □Moderate □Severe

3. Fatigue

0	1	2	3	4	5	6	7	8	9	10

None   Moderate   Always

4. Concentration Ability

0	1	2	3	4	5	6	7	8	9	10

None   Moderate   Always

5. Movement

0	1	2	3	4	5	6	7	8	9	10

Exercised   Couldn't Exercise

5. Aromatherapy Intervention

Aromatics Used	Route	□Room Diffusion for
1. ____________ 2. ____________ 3. ____________ 4. ____________	□Direct Inhalation □Topical to ________ body area at ______ %.	__________ minutes. □Other ________________

5. Post-Aromatherapy Level of Pain

0	1	2	3	4	5	6	7	8	9	10

No Pain   Moderate   Extreme Pain

2. Post-Aromatherapy Location(s) and Intensity of Pain

Head	Neck	Back	Shoulder	Arm	Glute	Hip	Leg
□None □Mild □Moderate □Severe	□None □Mild □Moderate □Severe	□None □Mild □Moderate □Severe	□None □Mild □Moderate □Severe	□None □Mild □Moderate □Severe	□None □Mild □Moderate □Severe	□None □Mild □Moderate □Severe	□None □Mild □Moderate □Severe

3. Post-Aromatherapy Fatigue

0	1	2	3	4	5	6	7	8	9	10

None   Moderate   Always

4. Post-Aromatherapy Concentration Ability

0	1	2	3	4	5	6	7	8	9	10

None   Moderate   Always

5. Post-Aromatherapy Movement

0	1	2	3	4	5	6	7	8	9	10

Exercised   Couldn't Exercise

Appendix B: Essential Oil Dilutions and Dosing

Topical: Skin Applications

Stage	Dose
Newborns to 3 months	0%
3 months to two years	0.25%
2-6 years	0.5-1%
6-15 years	0.5-1.5%
Adults	1.5-2.5%
Pregnancy/Breastfeeding	0.25-2%
Elders/Very Ill	0.25-1%
Acute Pain	5%

Carrier	0.25% dilution	0.5% dilution	1% dilution	2% dilution	3% dilution	5% dilution
5 mls			1 drop	2 drops	3 drops	5 drops
10 mls		1 drops	2 drops	4 drops	6 drops	10 drops
1 oz (30 mls)	1-2 drops	3 drops	6 drops	12 drops	18 drops	30 drops
2 ounce	3 drops	6 drops	12 drops	24 drops	36 drops	60 drops
3 ounce	4 drops	9 drops	18 drops	36 drops	54 drops	90 drops

Therapeutic Inhalation for Healthy Adults

TREATMENT	DOSE
Direct Inhalation - steam canopy, aromastick, or other device held directly to the nostrils	10 minutes
Indirect Inhalation - via diffuser in small room, application to the shower wall, during an aromatherapy massage	30 minutes
Environmental Fragrancing - via diffuser in large room, room spritzer, wall plug-in	30 minutes

Appendix B: Essential Oil Dilutions and Dosing. Adapted from *Clinical Aromatherapy for Health Professionals*, by Jane Buckle, 2006, R.J. Buckle Associates; *Aromatherapy in Midwifery Practice*, by Denise Tiran, 2016, Singing Dragon; and *Essential Oil Safety: A Guide for Health Care Professionals*, R. Tisserand & R. Young, 2014, Churchill Livingstone.

Appendix C: Resources

Recommended Texts:

I write book reviews pretty regularly over on Goodreads, you can find me here: https://www.goodreads.com/author/show/17136910.Amy_Kreydin. Books I think you'll enjoy reading include:

- Aromatherapy for Healing the Spirit – Gabriel Mojay
- Chemistry of Aromatherapeutic Oils, The – E. Joy Bowles
- Clinical Aromatherapy, Third Edition – Jane Buckle
- Complete Aromatherapy & Essential Oils, The – Purchon & Cantele
- Essential Oil Safety Second Edition – Tisserand & Young

Recommended Web Resources:

- American Botanical Council - studies, monographs – herbalgram.org
- AromaWeb - articles, recipes, essential oil profiles – aromaweb.com
- Cropwatch - "Independent watchdog for natural aromatics" – cropwatch.org

Professional Aromatherapy Associations

Use these organizations to find a qualified aromatherapist in your area.

- Alliance of International Aromatherapists (AIA) – aliance-aromatherapists.org
- Canadian Federation of Aromatherapists (CFA) – cfacanada.com
- International Aromatherapy & Aromatic Medicine Association (IAAMA) – iaama.org.au (Australia)
- International Federation of Professional Aromatherapists (IFPA) – ifparoma.org
- National Association for Holistic Aromatherapy (NAHA) – naha.org

References

- Abbas, A. K., Lichtman, A. H., & Pillai, S. (2016). Basic Immunology: Functions and Disorders of the Immune System. Fifth Edition. Elsevier.

- Aggarwal, B. B., Van Kuiken, M. E., Iyer, L. H., Harikumar, K. B., & Sung, B. (2009). Molecular targets of nutraceuticals derived from dietary spices: potential role in suppression of inflammation and tumorigenesis. *Experimental Biology and Medicine, 234*(8), 825-849.

- Alberts, B., Johnson, A., Lewis, J., Raff, M., Roberts, K., & Walter, P. (2002). *Molecular Biology of the Cell.*

- Ammon, H. P. T. (2016). Boswellic acids and their role in chronic inflammatory diseases. In *Anti-inflammatory Nutraceuticals and Chronic Diseases* (pp. 291-327). Springer, Cham.

- Anastasiou, C., & Buchbauer, G. Essential Oils as Immunomodulators: Some Examples. *Open Chemistry, 15*(1), 352-370.

- Bachmeier, B. E., Mohrenz, I. V., Mirisola, V., Schleicher, E., Romeo, F., Höhneke, C., & Pfeffer, U. (2007). Curcumin downregulates the inflammatory cytokines CXCL1 and-2 in breast cancer cells via NFκB. *Carcinogenesis, 29*(4), 779-789.

- Badria, F. A., El-Farahaty, T., Shabana, A. A., Hawas, S. A., & El-Batoty, M. F. (2002). Boswellia–curcumin preparation for treating knee osteoarthritis: a clinical evaluation. *Alternative & Complementary Therapies, 8*(6), 341-348.

- Basnet, P., & Skalko-Basnet, N. (2011). Curcumin: an anti-inflammatory molecule from a curry spice on the path to cancer treatment. *Molecules, 16*(6), 4567-4598.

- Berzins, S. P., Smyth, M. J., & Baxter, A. G. (2011). Presumed guilty: natural killer T cell defects and human disease. *Nature Reviews Immunology, 11*(2), 131.

- Blask, D. E. (2009). Melatonin, sleep disturbance and cancer risk. *Sleep Medicine Reviews, 13*(4), 257-264.

- Blum, S. (2013). The Immune System Recovery Plan: A Doctor's 4-step Program to Treat Autoimmune Disease. Simon and Schuster.

- Brandacher, G., Hoeller, E., Fuchs, D., & Weiss, H. G. (2007). Chronic immune activation underlies morbid obesity: is IDO a key player?. *Current Drug Metabolism, 8*(3), 289-295.

- Bryant, P. A., Trinder, J., & Curtis, N. (2004). Sick and tired: does sleep have a vital role in the immune system?. *Nature Reviews Immunology, 4*(6), 457.

- Buranen, M. (2013). Childhood trauma can cause illness in adulthood. *John Hopkins Magazine*, Winter 2013.

- Cantorna, M. T., Zhu, Y., Froicu, M., & Wittke, A. (2004). Vitamin D status, 1, 25-dihydroxyvitamin D3, and the immune system. *The American Journal of Clinical Nutrition, 80*(6), 1717S-1720S.

- Castanon-Cervantes, O., Wu, M., Ehlen, J. C., Paul, K., Gamble, K. L., Johnson, R. L., & Davidson, A. J. (2010). Dysregulation of inflammatory responses by chronic circadian disruption. *The Journal of Immunology, 185*(10), 5796-5805.

- Chopra, A., Lavin, P., Patwardhan, B., & Chitre, D. (2004). A 32-week randomized, placebo-controlled clinical evaluation of RA-11, an Ayurvedic drug, on osteoarthritis of the knees. *JCR: Journal of Clinical Rheumatology, 10*(5), 236-245.

- Cosentino, M., Luini, A., Bombelli, R., Corasaniti, M. T., Bagetta, G., & Marino, F. (2014). The essential oil of bergamot stimulates reactive oxygen species production in human polymorphonuclear leukocytes. *Phytotherapy research, 28*(8), 1232-1239.

- Dalgleish, A. G., & O'Byrne, K. J. (2002). Chronic immune activation and inflammation in the pathogenesis of AIDS and cancer. *Advances in Cancer Research,* 84, pg 231-276.

- Danese, A., & McEwen, B. S. (2012). Adverse childhood experiences, allostasis, allostatic load, and age-related disease. *Physiology & behavior, 106*(1), 29-39. Lappas, C. M., & Lappas, N. T. (2012). D-Limonene modulates T lymphocyte activity and viability. *Cellular Immunology, 279*(1), 30-41.

- Dantzer, R., O'Connor, J. C., Freund, G. G., Johnson, R. W., & Kelley, K. W. (2008). From inflammation to sickness and depression: when the immune system subjugates the brain. *Nature Reviews Neuroscience, 9*(1), 46.

- Dhabhar, F. S. (2009). Enhancing versus suppressive effects of stress on immune function: implications for immunoprotection and immunopathology. *Neuroimmunomodulation, 16*(5), 300-317.

- Diller, M. L., Kudchadkar, R. R., Delman, K. A., Lawson, D. H., & Ford, M. L. (2016). Balancing inflammation: the link between Th17 and regulatory T cells. *Mediators of Inflammation, 2016.*

- Donoyama, N., & Ichiman, Y. (2006). Which essential oil is better for hygienic massage practice?. *International Journal of Aromatherapy, 16*(3-4), 175-179.

- Donoyama, N., Wakuda, T., Tanitsu, T., & Ichiman, Y. (2005). Using tea tree oil for hygienic massage practice. *International Journal of Aromatherapy, 15*(2), 106-109.

- Dube, S. R., Fairweather, D., Pearson, W. S., Felitti, V. J., Anda, R. F., & Croft, J. B. (2009). Cumulative childhood stress and autoimmune diseases in adults. *Psychosomatic Medicine, 71*(2), 243.

- Elenkov, I. J., Webster, E. L., Torpy, D. J., & Chrousos, G. P. (1999). Stress, corticotropin-releasing hormone, glucocorticoids, and the immune/inflammatory response: acute and chronic effects. *Annals of the New York Academy of Sciences, 876*(1), 1-13.

- Fogel, L. A., Yokoyama, W. M., & French, A. R. (2013). Natural killer cells in human autoimmune disorders. *Arthritis Research & Therapy, 15*(4), 216.

- Fortes, M. B., Diment, B. C., Di Felice, U., & Walsh, N. P. (2012). Dehydration decreases saliva antimicrobial proteins important for mucosal immunity. *Applied Physiology, Nutrition, and Metabolism, 37*(5), 850-859.

- Gamaldo, C. E., Shaikh, A. K., & McArthur, J. C. (2012). The sleep-immunity relationship. *Neurologic Clinics, 30*(4), 1313-1343.

- Gerhardt, H., Seifert, F., Buvari, P., Vogelsang, H., & Repges, R. (2001).

Therapie des aktiven Morbus Crohn mit dem Boswellia-serrata-Extrakt H 15. *Zeitschrift für Gastroenterologie, 39*(01), 11-17.

- Gerra, G., Monti, D., Panerai, A. E., Sacerdote, P., Anderlini, R., Avanzini, P., & Franceschi, C. (2003). Long-term immune-endocrine effects of bereavement: relationships with anxiety levels and mood. *Psychiatry Research, 121*(2), 145-158.

- Glaser, R., & Kiecolt-Glaser, J. K. (1998). Stress-associated immune modulation: relevance to viral infections and chronic fatigue syndrome. *The American Journal of Medicine, 105*(3), 35S-42S.

- Grice, E. A., Kong, H. H., Conlan, S., Deming, C. B., Davis, J., Young, A. C.,. & Turner, M. L. (2009). Topographical and temporal diversity of the human skin microbiome. *Science*, 324(5931), 1190-1192.

- Grossmann, M. E., Mizuno, N. K., Schuster, T., & Cleary, M. P. (2010). Punicic acid is an ω-5 fatty acid capable of inhibiting breast cancer proliferation. *International Journal of Oncology 36*(2), 421-426.

- Gupta, I., Gupta, V., Parihar, A., Gupta, S., Lüdtke, R., Safayhi, H., & Ammon, H. P. (1998). Effects of Boswellia serrata gum resin in patients with bronchial asthma: results of a double-blind, placebo-controlled, 6-week clinical study. *European Journal of Medical Research, 3*(11), 511-514.

- Gupta, I., Parihar, A., Malhotra, P., Gupta, S., Lüdtke, R., Safayhi, H., & Ammon, H. P. (2001). Effects of gum resin of Boswellia serrata in patients with chronic colitis. *Planta Medica, 67*(05), 391-395.

- Harvard Women's Health Watch. (June, 2014). Foods that fight inflammation: Doctors are learning that one of the best ways to quell inflammation lies not in the medicine cabinet, but in the refrigerator. *Harvard Health Publishing*. Retrieved from https://www.health.harvard.edu/staying-healthy/foods-that-fight-inflammation.

- Hwang, J. H. (2006). The effects of the inhalation method using essential oils on blood pressure and stress responses of clients with essential hypertension. *Journal of Korean Academy of Nursing, 36*(7), 1123-1134.

- Huxley, R. R., Ansary-Moghaddam, A., Clifton, P., Czernichow, S., Parr, C. L., & Woodward, M. (2009). The impact of dietary and lifestyle risk factors on risk of colorectal cancer: a quantitative overview of the epidemiological evidence. *International Journal of Cancer, 125*(1), 171-180.

- Institute of Medicine. 2005. Dietary Reference Intakes for Water, Potassium, Sodium, Chloride, and Sulfate. Washington, DC: The National Academies Press.

- Irwin, M. (2002). Psychoneuroimmunology of depression: clinical implications. *Brain, Behavior, and Immunity,* Vol: 16, Issue: 1, Page: 1-16.

- Karlberg, A. T., Magnusson, K., & Nilsson, U. (1992). Air oxidation of d-limonene (the citrus solvent) creates potent allergens. *Contact Dermatitis, 26*(5), 332-340.

- Kiecolt-Glaser, J. K., Robles, T. F., Heffner, K. L., Loving, T. J., & Glaser, R. (2002). Psycho-oncology and cancer: psychoneuroimmunology and cancer. *Annals of Oncology, 13*(suppl_4), 165-169.

- Koeppen, K. (2013). Frankincense Fears Largely Unfounded. *National Association for Holistic Aromatherapy*. Retrieved from https://naha.org/naha-blog/frankincense-fears-largely-unfounded

- Kong, H. H., & Segre, J. A. (2012). Skin microbiome: looking back to move forward. Journal of Investigative Dermatology, 132(3), 933-939.

- Kong, H. H., Oh, J., Deming, C., Conlan, S., Grice, E. A., Beatson, M. A., & Turner, M. L. (2012). Temporal shifts in the skin microbiome associated with disease flares and treatment in children with atopic dermatitis. Genome research, 22(5), 850-859.

- Kuriyama, H., Watanabe, S., Nakaya, T., Shigemori, I., Kita, M., Yoshida, N., & Imanishi, J. (2005). Immunological and psychological benefits of aromatherapy massage. *Evidence-Based Complementary and Alternative Medicine, 2*(2), 179-184.

- Lai, P. K., & Roy, J. (2004). Antimicrobial and chemopreventive properties of herbs and spices. *Current Medicinal Chemistry, 11*(11), 1451-1460.

- Lampe, J. W. (2003). Spicing up a vegetarian diet: chemopreventive effects of phytochemicals. *The American Journal of Clinical Nutrition, 78*(3), 579S-583S.

- Li, Q., Otsuka, T., Kobayashi, M., Wakayama, Y., Inagaki, H., Katsumata, M., & Suzuki, H. (2011). Acute effects of walking in forest environments on cardiovascular and metabolic parameters. *European Journal of Applied Physiology, 111*(11), 2845-2853.

- Li, X. J., Yang, Y. J., Li, Y. S., Zhang, W. K., & Tang, H. B. (2016). α-Pinene, linalool, and 1-octanol contribute to the topical anti-inflammatory and analgesic activities of frankincense by inhibiting COX-2. *Journal of Ethnopharmacology, 179*, 22-26.

- Liju, V. B., Jeena, K., & Kuttan, R. (2011). An evaluation of antioxidant, anti-inflammatory, and antinociceptive activities of essential oil from Curcuma longa. L. *Indian Journal of Pharmacology, 43*(5), 526.

- Lillehei, A. S., & Halcon, L. L. (2014). A systematic review of the effect of inhaled essential oils on sleep. *The Journal of Alternative and Complementary Medicine, 20*(6), 441-451.

- Madisch, A., Miehlke, S., Eichele, O., Mrwa, J., Bethke, B., Kuhlisch, E., ... & Stolte, M. (2007). Boswellia serrata extract for the treatment of collagenous colitis. A double-blind, randomized, placebo-controlled, multicenter trial. *International Journal of Colorectal Disease, 22*(12), 1445-1451.

- Manuele, M. G., Ferraro, G., & Anesini, C. (2008). Effect of Tilia× viridis flower extract on the proliferation of a lymphoma cell line and on normal murine lymphocytes: contribution of monoterpenes, especially limonene. *Phytotherapy Research, 22*(11), 1520-1526.

- Martineau, A. R., Jolliffe, D. A., Hooper, R. L., Greenberg, L., Aloia, J. F., Bergman, P., & Goodall, E. C. (2017). Vitamin D supplementation to prevent acute respiratory tract infections: systematic review and meta-analysis of individual participant data. BMJ, *356*, i6583.

- Marin, T. J., Chen, E., Munch, J. A., & Miller, G. E. (2009). Double-exposure to acute stress and chronic family stress is associated with immune changes in children with asthma. Psychosomatic Medicine, 71(4), 378.

- Matura, M., Goossens, A., Bordalo, O., Garcia-Bravo, B., Magnussona, K., Wrangsjö, K., & Karlberg, A. T. (2002). Oxidized citrus oil (R-limonene): a frequent skin sensitizer in Europe. Journal of the American Academy of Dermatology, 47(5), 709-714.

- Matura, M., Sköld, M., Börje, A., Andersen, K. E., Bruze, M., Frosch, P., & Karlberg, A. T. (2006). Not only oxidized R-(+)-but also S-(−)-limonene is a common cause of contact allergy in dermatitis patients in Europe. Contact Dermatitis, 55(5), 274-279.

- Michaud, D. S., Spiegelman, D., Clinton, S. K., Rimm, E. B., Curhan, G. C., Willett, W. C., & Giovannucci, E. L. (1999). Fluid intake and the risk of bladder cancer in men. *New England Journal of Medicine, 340*(18), 1390-1397.

- Moretti, M. D., Peana, A. T., & Satta, M. (1997). A study on anti-inflammatory and peripheral analgesic action of Salvia sclarea oil and its main components. *Journal of Essential Oil Research, 9*(2), 199-204.

- O'Byrne, K. J., & Dalgleish, A. G. (2001). Chronic immune activation and inflammation as the cause of malignancy. *British Journal of Cancer, 85*(4), 473.

- Peana, A. T., D'Aquila, P. S., Panin, F., Serra, G., Pippia, P., & Moretti, M. D. L. (2002). Anti-inflammatory activity of linalool and linalyl acetate constituents of essential oils. *Phytomedicine, 9*(8), 721-726.

- Pole, S. (2006). Ayurvedic medicine: the principles of traditional practice. Elsevier Health Sciences.

- Rook, G. A., & Lowry, C. A. (2008). The hygiene hypothesis and psychiatric disorders. *Trends in immunology, 29*(4), 150-158.

- Rossi, T., Melegari, M., Bianchi, A., Albasini, A., & Vampa, G. (1988). Sedative, anti-inflammatory and anti-diuretic effects induced in rats by essential oils of varieties of Anthemis nobilis: a comparative study. *Pharmacological Research Communications, 20*, 71-74.

- Santos, F. A., & Rao, V. S. N. (2000). Antiinflammatory and antinociceptive effects of 1, 8-cineole a terpenoid oxide present in many plant essential oils. *Phytotherapy Research, 14*(4), 240-244.

- Schleifer, S. J., Keller, S. E., Camerino, M., Thornton, J. C., & Stein, M. (1983). Suppression of lymphocyte stimulation following bereavement. *JAMA, 250*(3), 374-377.

- Shannon, J., White, E., Shattuck, A. L., & Potter, J. D. (1996). Relationship of food groups and water intake to colon cancer risk. *Cancer Epidemiology and Prevention Biomarkers, 5*(7), 495-502.

- Sherer, M. L., Posillico, C. K., & Schwarz, J. M. (2017). The psychoneuroimmunology of pregnancy. *Frontiers in Neuroendocrinology*.

- Sigurdardottir, L. G., Valdimarsdottir, U. A., Mucci, L. A., Fall, K., Rider, J. R., Schernhammer, E., ... & Gudnason, V. (2013). Sleep disruption among older men and risk of prostate cancer. Cancer Epidemiology and Prevention

Biomarkers, 22(5), 872-879.

- Silva, J., Abebe, W., Sousa, S. M., Duarte, V. G., Machado, M. I. L., & Matos, F. J. A. (2003). Analgesic and anti-inflammatory effects of essential oils of Eucalyptus. *Journal of ethnopharmacology, 89*(2-3), 277-283.

- Smith, L. L. (2003). Overtraining, excessive exercise, and altered immunity. *Sports Medicine, 33*(5), 347-364.

- Sontakke, S., Thawani, V., Pimpalkhute, S., Kabra, P., Babhulkar, S., & Hingorani, L. (2007). Open, randomized, controlled clinical trial of Boswellia serrata extract as compared to valdecoxib in osteoarthritis of knee. *Indian Journal of Pharmacology, 39*(1), 27.

- Standen, M. D., Connellan, P. A., & Leach, D. N. (2006). Natural killer cell activity and lymphocyte activation: Investigating the effects of a selection of essential oils and components in vitro. *International Journal of Aromatherapy, 16*(3-4), 133-139.

- Stern, R. S. (2010). Prevalence of a history of skin cancer in 2007: results of an incidence-based model. *Archives of Dermatology, 146*(3), 279-282.

- Stevens, C. D., & Miller, L. E. (2016). *Clinical Immunology and Serology: A Laboratory Perspective.* FA Davis.

- Stratton, S. P., Stratton, M. S., & Alberts, D. S. (2006). Promising agents for chemoprevention of skin cancer. *Current Oncology, 13*(5), 185.

- Strickland, I., Rhodes, L. E., Flanagan, B. F., & Friedmann, P. S. (1997). TNF-α and IL-8 are upregulated in the epidermis of normal human skin after UVB exposure: correlation with neutrophil accumulation and E-selectin expression. *Journal of Investigative Dermatology, 108*(5), 763-768.

- Stürner, K. H., Stellmann, J. P., Dörr, J., Paul, F., Friede, T., Schammler, S., & Werz, O. (2017). A standardised frankincense extract reduces disease activity in relapsing-remitting multiple sclerosis (the SABA phase IIa trial). *J Neurol Neurosurg Psychiatry*, jnnp-2017.

- Takaki, I., Bersani-Amado, L. E., Vendruscolo, A., Sartoretto, S. M., Diniz, S. P., Bersani-Amado, C. A., & Cuman, R. K. N. (2008). Anti-inflammatory and antinociceptive effects of Rosmarinus officinalis L. essential oil in experimental animal models. *Journal of medicinal food, 11*(4), 741-746.

- Thompson, C. L., Larkin, E. K., Patel, S., Berger, N. A., Redline, S., & Li, L. (2011). Short duration of sleep increases risk of colorectal adenoma. Cancer, 117(4), 841-847.

- Thompson, C. L., & Li, L. (2012). Association of sleep duration and breast cancer OncotypeDX recurrence score. Breast cancer research and treatment, 134(3), 1291-1295.

- Tisserand, R., & Young, R. (2014). *Essential Oil Safety: A Guide for Health Care Professionals.* Churchill Livingstone 2014.

- Tsai, M. L., Lin, C. C., Lin, W. C., & Yang, C. H. (2011). Antimicrobial, antioxidant, and anti-inflammatory activities of essential oils from five selected herbs. *Bioscience, Biotechnology, and Biochemistry, 75*(10), 1977-1983.

- Verma, R., Foster, R. E., Horgan, K., Mounsey, K., Nixon, H., Smalle, N., ... & Carter, C. R. (2016). Lymphocyte depletion and repopulation after chemotherapy for primary breast cancer. *Breast Cancer Research, 18*(1), 10.

- Vishteh, A., Thomas, I., & Imamura, T. (1986). Eugenol modulation of the immune response in mice. *Immunopharmacology, 12*(3), 187-192.

- Waugh, A., & Grant, A. (2010). Ross & Wilson Anatomy and Physiology in Health and Illness E-Book. Elsevier Health Sciences.

- Wieten, L., van der Zee, R., Spiering, R., Wagenaar-Hilbers, J., van Kooten, P. J., Broere, F., & van Eden, W. (2009). The oregano constituent carvacrol boosts stress protein Hsp70 to activate T cell regulation of inflammation in autoimmune arthritis. *Endogenous stress proteins as targets for anti-inflammatory T cells*, 125.

- Zhao, B., Li, X., He, R., Cheng, S., & Wenjuan, X. (1989). Scavenging effect of extracts of green tea and natural antioxidants on active oxygen radicals. *Cell biophysics, 14*(2), 175-185.

- Zhou, H. L., Deng, Y. M., & Xie, Q. M. (2006). The modulatory effects of the volatile oil of ginger on the cellular immune response in vitro and in vivo in mice. *Journal of ethnopharmacology, 105*(1-2), 301-305.

- Ziemssen, T., & Kern, S. (2007). Psychoneuroimmunology–cross-talk between the immune and nervous systems. *Journal of Neurology, 254*(2), II8-II11.

Dear Reader

Thank you for reading *Aromatic Immunity*! I hope you found this volume helpful in navigating research on using aromatics that influence the immune system. If you did, consider helping me spread the word! You can help others find this book by writing reviews, a blog post, or talking about it on your social media pages. Reviews and shares help writers like me keep writing, and I appreciate your support! You hold the power to help others find out more about this important topic in aromatherapy.

Thank you,
Amy Kreydin

Want more? Join me on Facebook at fb.com/barefootdragonfly for articles, tips, recipes, and events (online and here in Central Texas).

Acknowledgements

"If I have seen further it is by standing on the shoulders of giants."
- Sir Isaac Newton

I am deeply grateful to the intellectual giants who have generously leant me the use of their shoulders so that I might become a better wellness practitioner, and a more thoughtful researcher. They include Kathy Duffy – for cultivating my foundation in Clinical Aromatherapy; Mark Webb – for a brilliant introduction to Aromatic Medicine; Rhiannon Lewis – for providing gentle guidance on challenging case studies over the years; Robert Tisserand – for inspiring confidence in research and introducing me to the fascinating world of biofilms; Sylla Sheppard-Hangar – for being an energetic cheerleader, offering encouragement and support with no strings attached; Peter Holmes – for expanding my understanding of fragrance energetics; Gabriel Mojay – for fostering learning environments; and Marco Valusi – for brilliant breakdowns of aromatic chemistry.

My deepest thanks to colleagues and peers, who have brainstormed case studies with me, encouraged me through this writing project, and have otherwise offered support as my career as a clinical aromatherapist and board certified reflexologist has evolved. I'd especially like to thank Lauren Bridges – for her invaluable insight on case studies and formulations; Nyssa Rhiannon Hanger – for helping me hone my theories on aromatics for chronic inflammation and HPV; Katharine Koeppen – for sharing her clinical expertise on case studies; Sue Pace – for her clinical expertise on drug interactions; Ann Fuller – for always being game to geek out on the mind-immune connection with me; Ken Miller – for pharmacology input on case studies and theories; Hana Bělíková – for encouraging me at each step of this book; Madeleine Kerkhof – for encouragement to write on this subject and the amazing oregano blossom and butterfly image on the cover; Li Wong – for encouragement and valuable input in writing this book; Kayla Fioravanti – for encouragement in writing this book.

Thank you to my husband, Oleg, who has supported me in all of my Barefoot Dragonfly endeavors over the years, including this project. For your tireless cheerleading, reminders for me to eat when I get lost in writing and research, and being my 'math guy' when I need help sorting out a formula, thank you. This book could not have happened without you, Babe!

I am very grateful to my students and clients who have peppered me with questions, trusted me to be part of their wellness teams, and otherwise given me the opportunity to write a book based on these experiences.

Thank you to my parents, who nurtured my love of plants and wellness from a young age, and who have been willing test subjects for a myriad aromatic remedies.

A huge thank you to my proofreaders Tess Clark and Lauren Bridges, you ladies rock!

Thank you to my local and distance team of allied health practitioner, who have helped me better understand autoimmunity and chronic inflammation, and approaches to wellness.

And thanks go to you, reader, for supporting me through the purchase of this book. I hope you've found new approaches to your wellness plan.

Gratefully Yours,
Amy Kreydin

Books by Amy Kreydin

Aromatic Waters: Therapeutic, Cosmetic, and Culinary Hydrosol Applications (2017)

Friends Don't Let Friends Drink Essential Oils (2017)

Aromatic Immunity: Navigating Essential Oil Research for Cancer, Autoimmune, and Chronic Inflammatory Conditions (2018)

Classes by Amy Kreydin

200-Hour Aromatherapy Certificate Course

300-Hour Reflexology Certificate Course

Aromatic Therapies in the Childbearing Year

Introduction to Hydrosols

A Holistic Approach to Pain Management

A Functional Clinical Aromatherapy Approach to SIBO

Aromatic Beauty Care – Apothecary Session

Sippable Botanicals: Drinking Vinegars

Foot and Hand Spa – Apothecary Session

Supporting the Immune System – Apothecary Session

Achoo! Aromatic Support for Allergies

Ayurvedic Self-Care Foot Rub Class

www.thebarefootdragonfly.com